Kettlebells

Lose the Fat and Get Fit with Kettlebells

The information herein is offered for informational purposes solely, and is universal as so. The presentation of the information is without contract or any type of guarantee assurance.

The trademarks that are used are without any consent, and the publication of the trademark is without permission or backing by the trademark owner. All trademarks and brands within this book are for clarifying purposes only and are the owned by the owners themselves, not affiliated with this document.

Contents

Introduction

Kettlebells have become a gym staple today because of the unlimited training opportunities they offer. A kettlebell is a type of dumbbell except that the weight is not distributed evenly in a kettlebell. Kettlebells are shaped like a ball that comes with a handle to provide an easy grip. Kettlebells can range from 5 pounds to over 100 pounds in weight.

Kettlebell training has become a popular method to lose weight, build strength, improve balance, maintain fitness, and get a toned and beautiful body. Kettlebell training has now become a part of most of the weight loss programs because it is a time-saving calorie burning solution. According to the American Council on Exercise (ACE), an average person can burn <u>400 calories in just twenty minutes</u> by doing kettlebell exercises.

The origin of kettlebells is still a matter of speculation. The word 'Girya' meaning kettlebell was first published in the Russian dictionary in the early eighteenth century. Kettlebells became popular in the West in the late twentieth century when a Soviet physical training instructor wrote an article on Kettlebells in a popular American magazine.

There are many different weight loss exercises that can be done with kettlebells. Some of the most popular ones include the following:

1. Air squat

2. Kettlebell deadlift

3. Kettlebell goblet squat

4. Kettlebell two-handed swing

5. Kettlebell one-handed swing

Some of these exercises require high degree of training and skill. If not done properly, kettlebell exercises may provide little benefit and can result in serious injuries. Guidance by a qualified trainer can help the user in having a safe and effective experience of kettlebell exercises.

What are Kettlebells?

Kettlebells are a kind of free weights, shaped like a ball with a handle to provide easy grip. There is a handle at one end of the iron-cast ball, which results in an uneven distribution of weight. The unbalanced distribution of weight results in a more extensive work out of the muscles in order to stabilize and maintain balance and counteract the momentum.

Kettlebells generally come in standardized weight of 35 pounds, but can range from 5 pounds to over 100 pounds. Kettlebells are small and portable; therefore, they can be incorporated in all types of fitness and athletic trainings.

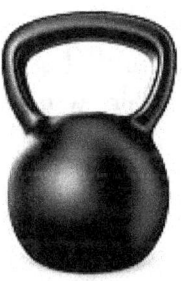

Material of the Kettlebells

Kettlebells are usually made up of cast-iron but some kettlebells are coated with other materials like vinyl or rubber. The cast-iron kettlebell is also called the 'original' kettlebell and is most frequently used. The vinyl-coated kettlebell is essentially similar to the original kettlebell but it contains a coating of vinyl over the ball and handle of the kettlebell, which gives it a more sophisticated look. Rubber-coated kettlebells are not prone to rust or get scratches.

Cast-iron kettlebells come in black color only. Vinyl-coated kettlebells can be made in any color. The performance of cast-iron kettlebell and vinyl-coated kettlebell does not differ a lot. Vinyl-coated kettlebells may grab the skin uncomfortably in certain exercise positions.

Types of Kettlebells

There are two variations available in kettlebells, the original kettlebells and the competition kettlebells.

Original Kettlebells

Original kettlebells consist of a ball and a rounded handle made up of cast-iron. The diameter of the ball may vary based on the weight of the ball and the manufacturer. This type of kettlebell is used by people who are interested in general fitness training.

Competition Kettlebells

Competition kettlebells or Pro Grade Kettlebells are used by individuals who are kettlebell fanatics or are involved in kettlebell sport. They are more durable as compared to cast-iron kettlebells because they are made of high-grade steel. These kettlebells come with a square-shaped handle. The diameter of the ball remains constant regardless of the weight of the kettlebell. This means that whether you are using a 16 pound kettlebell or an 8 pound kettlebell, it will rest on the exact same place on your forearm. Competition kettlebells have a thinner handle to provide a lasting grip and to minimize fatigue with strenuous repetition sets.

The History of Kettlebells

Ancient History of Kettlebells

The history of kettlebells is somewhat unclear but there is archeological evidence that Kettlebells were used for strength building in ancient Greece. A kettlebell weighing 143 kg is stored in the Archaeological Museum of Olympia, Athens, Greece.

Russian Origin of Kettlebells

The word kettlebell appeared first time in 1704 in a Russian dictionary. At that time, 'Girya' or Kettlebell was only used in measuring weight of grains and other goods. The use of kettlebells in physical training had not started until the late eighteenth century.

The founder of heavy athletics, Dr. Vladislav Kraevsky, travelled through the Europe from 1870 to 1880 in order to gather information about physical sports and finding new ways to improve physical health. He introduced the Russian athletes to exercises that involved dumbbells and kettlebells.

The origin of weightlifting in Russia dates back to 1885 when Dr. Kraevsky founded a weight training hall with the goal of muscle development of Russian athletes. The kettlebells continued to flourish in Russia but their spread to other parts of the world was restricted by the World War I and the Russian civil war.

The Russian government aimed to minimize country's health care expenses by making kettlebell training mandatory for the public. The Russian armed forces also started using Kettlebells sports as a measure of soldiers' physical strength. By 1974, kettlebell sport had been officially declared as the ethnic sport of Russia.

Kettlebells' Journey to the West

Kettlebells were not introduced in the West until the late twentieth century when a Russian physical training instructor wrote an article on Kettlebells in a popular American athletes' magazine. Inspired with the benefits of kettlebells, the Dragon Door Publications decided to start manufacturing Kettlebells in America. They approached the Russian instructor and requested him to teach American people how to use the kettlebells.

In 2002, kettlebells' popularity took off when it made it into the Rolling Stone Magazine as 'the hot weight of the year'.

Girevoy Sport

Kettlebell lifting or kettlebell sport, which is called Girevoy sport in Russian language, has a long history in Russia. In 1948, the first kettlebell competition was held in which 55 athletes took part. The athletes, who were called Gireviks, competed in kettlebell sports in three disciplines with no time limits; the press, the snatch, and the jerk.

The kettlebell sports modern history started in 1962 when rules were unified and time limits were enforced. Kettlebell lifting further gained popularity in 1985 when the first championship of the Soviet Union was organized and winner was given the title of 'Master of Sports'.

The first European championship took place in 1992, which was organized by the European Union of Weightball Lifting. In 1993, a world championship was held in which 96 athletes from 5 different countries participated. Women were allowed to take part in Kettlebell lifting in 1999.

How Does a Kettlebell Help You Lose Weight?

Kettlebells are one of the simplest and most effective weight loss tools around. The weight of a kettlebell is centered below the handle, so it needs a lot of energy and muscle work to counteract the momentum. There are many reasons to why kettlebells are becoming the most popular choice of weight loss.

Burn More Calories in Less Time

Kettlebells are different from traditional free weights because traditional weights aim at certain muscle groups only and rest of the body muscles remain static. Kettlebell training is very demanding; it does not isolate muscle groups and gets your whole body moving. This results in much more oxygen and energy requirement and leads to burning of huge amounts of fat in a very short span of time.

Burn Calories Even After Training

Excessive post-exercise oxygen consumption (EPOC) or Afterburn refers to the loss of calories that occurs after training due to increased metabolic rate of the body. Kettlebells can produce an afterburn effect that may last for more than 24 hours.

During an extensive training session, the muscles' demand for oxygen increases creating an oxygen shortage, and causes the body to ask for more oxygen after training. More oxidation results in more fat breakdown which causes weight loss.

Kettlebell exercises are high-intensity exercises. High-intensity exercises result in lactic acid accumulation in muscles and depletion of body's oxygen stores. As a result, the body is forced to work harder in order to replenish the oxygen stores for a period of 24 to 36 hours post-training.

Which Kettlebell is Right for You?

Picking the right kettlebell is essential in order to get the most out of kettlebell training and to avoid injuries. The selection of a kettlebell depends on various factors such as type of training, age, gender, weight, fitness level, and previous experience with kettlebells.

Type of Training

There are many different types of kettlebell exercises; generally we can divide those kettlebell movements into two categories:

Ballistic Lifts

Ballistic lifts include kettlebell swings, snatches, judging, and tossing. Ballistic lifts usually require a heavier kettlebell but beginners should not put a lot of stress on themselves because strength building with kettlebells takes time; therefore, it is better to start with a lighter kettlebell and perform the exercises effectively before moving on to a heavier kettlebell.

Kettlebell Grinds

Grinding movements include get-ups, windmills, overhead presses, and bent press, which result in constant tension on the muscles and a greater chance of muscle injury. Grinding movements require attention to whole-body tension and regulation of sustained power breathing; therefore, these exercises are usually done with a smaller kettlebell.

Gender

Kettlebell choices for men and women are different because of the difference in their body strengths. Generally, it is seen that women tend to choose lighter kettlebells, whereas men over-estimate their strength and end up choosing a kettlebell too heavy to endure. Starting kettlebell weight for men and women is different and depends on their level of fitness and type of training.

Kettlebell Sizes for Men

Kettlebell training is technical and requires a lot of strength and experience. Therefore, choosing a kettlebell size that is reasonable to start with is important.

12 - 16 KG – Men with very little strength and small-build are advised to start with a kettlebell of 12kg to 16kg. Individuals with medium-build who had recent rehabilitation from injuries or have low fitness level and experience with kettlebell can also start with similar weights.

16 - 20 KG: Kettlebells of 16-20kg are best suited for men of medium build with average strength and fitness level.

20 - 24 KG – Strong, athletic, active men with an extensive training experience and high fitness level can start with a kettlebell of 20-24kg.

The choice of kettlebell is also affected by the type of training. For ballistic movements, average-build active men should start with a 16kg or a 20kg kettlebell. Athletic men with medium to large build can start with a kettlebell of 16kg or 28kg.

For grinding movements, choose a kettlebell that you can easily press overhead about eight to ten times. Active men can start with an 8kg kettlebell, while athletic men can choose a kettlebell of 12kg.

Kettlebell Sizes for Women

For women, starting weight of kettlebell depends on their current level of fitness and exercises that they intend to perform with it.

8 - 12 KG – This is the ideal weight to start with for most women, especially for those who have small build, very little training experience, and who have undergone recent rehabilitation from injuries.

12 - 16 KG – Women with average build and little strength training experience can start kettlebell training with a 12kg or a 16kg kettlebell.

16 - 20 kg – Women who have an extensive strength training experience, very good cardiovascular fitness, and strong build can start with a 16kg or a 20kg kettlebell under the supervision of an experienced instructor.

For ballistic movements, inactive women should start with a 6kg or an 8kg kettlebell. An 8kg kettlebell is the most popular starting weight for women who are active but new to kettlebell training. Athletic women can start with a 12kg kettlebell also.

For grinding movements, inactive women should start with a 4kg kettlebell. An average, active woman can start with a kettlebell of 8kg and athletic women can start with a 12kg kettlebell.

What Type of Kettlebell Should You Choose?

There are different types of kettlebells available in the market. You should select a kettlebell that suits your needs and your body structure. There are certain attributes that should be kept in mind in order to select a good quality kettlebell.

Smooth Curved Handle

Quality kettlebells come with a smooth, curved handle that can be grasped anywhere. Do not select a kettlebell that has an angular or squarish angle. The handle should be round and wide enough to allow you to hold it with both hands side by side when doing two handed kettlebells. If you are selecting a vinyl-coated or a painted kettlebell, make sure that the paint is of good quality. Good quality paint would not chip, crack, or rust easily and the pristine look of your kettlebell will be maintained for a long time.

Thickness of the kettlebell handle is also an important consideration. Improper thickness of handle can place you in danger of dropping the kettlebell and injuring yourself. An improper thin grip is when you hold the handle and your fingers are meeting the palm. An improper thick grip is when you hold the hand and your fingers are too far apart. Ideally, your fingers should be one and a half inches from the palm when holding the kettlebell.

Handle to ball gap is important for pressing exercises. If it is too short or long, the kettlebell will not fall in the right spot during certain exercises. The ideal gap between handle and ball should be about two and a half inches.

A Flat Base

Look for a kettlebell that has a flat base so that it can rest on the floor without tilting. Rubber-coated kettlebells are also available but they can be unsuitable for certain exercises and when dropped it may bounce back and hit you. Rubber-coated kettlebells are easier on the floor and cause little damage to the floor when dropped accidently.

Stated Weight

It is important to check that there is no variation in the stated weight and actual weight of the kettlebell. Inexpensive kettlebells that are manufactured by untrustworthy companies may have a huge variation in their weights. So, it is better to stick with reputable companies only when selecting a kettlebell.

Kettlebell Assembling

There are two basic methods to make a kettlebell: One piece casting and two piece assembly. In two piece assembly, a handle is attached to the ball and as a result this kettlebell is not as strong and secure as a kettlebell made by one-piece casting method. The heavy ball of a kettlebell constructed using two piece assembly method may get separated from the handle during a swing and cause injury.

How to Know if You Have Chosen the Right Size?

It is important to test a kettlebell before purchasing it. There are three basic exercises that can help you to figure out if you have chosen the right size of kettlebell or not.

1. Place the kettlebell in one hand and lift it above your head. If you are able to lift your arm without arching your back and hold up the kettlebell for a few seconds then it is right for you.

2. Hold the kettlebell with both hands between your legs with your feet slightly wider than hip-distance apart. Bend your knees and swing the kettlebell. If you are able to straighten your legs without any pain and lift the kettlebell above shoulder's height then the kettlebell size is appropriate.

3. Hold the handle of kettlebell with both hands while standing with your feet hip-distance apart. Squat down and swing the kettlebell in between your legs. If you are able to straighten your legs without your back or shoulders hurting then the kettlebell size is appropriate for you.

Alternatives to a Kettlebell

Kettlebells can be pricey and hard to find. Even if you own a kettlebell, you cannot have it with you all the time such as while travelling or when you do not have access to gym. Some people use regular free weights such as dumbbells to perform kettlebell exercises but they are not as effective as a kettlebell. Working out with a dumbbell does not challenge your balance the same way as a kettlebell does because in kettlebells weight is concentrated in the middle, not on either side. A better cheap alternative to kettlebells is to use household containers to create a less pricey version of kettlebell.

You can use a plastic gallon filled with water, sand, salt, or gravel in place of a kettlebell. A one gallon container filled with water weighs around 8.5 pounds, which is not enough for many kettlebell exercises such as chest press. A two gallon container packed with sand or gravel weighs a respectable amount around 15 to 20 pounds, which is enough for a beginner or an intermediate workout.

It is important to test your container or jug for cracks or leaks before beginning your kettlebell training. Even with a screw cap little leakage can occur. You may use glue or duct tape to seal the opening or use a more durable container like a gas can.

Kettlebell Exercises

Kettlebell Goblet Squat

The kettlebell goblet squat is a lower body exercise that develops strength of quadriceps femoris muscles and calf muscles. Unlike the traditional squats, it is done by keeping the body in an erect position that results in lesser strain on the spine and lower lumbar. Holding the kettlebell in front shifts your center of gravity, which tightens up your trunk and abs in order to brace the weight.

The Kettlebell Goblet Squat can be done in two ways. One way is using a heavier kettlebell with fewer repetitions that causes tears in the muscle fiber and cause them to grow thicker and stronger. Another method involves high work rate with low repetitions forcing more and more oxygenated blood into the hamstrings, quadriceps, and glutes.

The goblet squat can be performed using dumbbells, medicine balls, sandbags, and other free weights, but the kettlebell is perfectly designed for the goblet squat because it shifts your center of gravity allowing you to exert more force. Also, kettlebells come with handles so you can hold it nice and contained against your chest.

How to do a Kettlebell Goblet Squat

1. Stand up straight holding the kettlebell by its handle at your chest height.

2. Slowly descend into a squat position keeping your head and chest up and maintaining your back in a straight position until your hamstrings are touching your calves.

3. Pause briefly at this position and then move upwards concentrating the force on your legs and not on your back.

Tips to Perform Kettlebell Goblet Squat Correctly

Throughout the movement, the kettlebell and your arms should not move and all the movement should come from your legs. Keep your back straight and your abs locked, do not arch your back or bend forward. Your elbows should remain between your knees. Heels and toes should remain planted on the floor and the hips should ascend at the same rate as the shoulders. Never perform kettlebell goblet squat in bare feet because in case the kettlebell is dropped it can cause fractures.

Video: https://youtu.be/mvVPrpusmrk

Kettlebell Squat

Kettlebell squat is the most basic exercise to familiarize an individual with kettlebell training. Squat is a basic human movement, which is used often in everyday tasks such as sitting in a chair. Squat is an essential for kettlebell training. Regular squats improve posture, mobility, and strengthen the lower body.

Holding a kettlebell while doing squats can target your arms, shoulders, and abs muscles. Kettlebell squats are great for weight loss and strength building. This exercise is designed to mobilize your large muscle groups, which include quadriceps, glutes, and hamstrings. Kettlebell squats are also called Kettlebell front squats because weight is in front of you unlike traditional squats in which force is exerted across your shoulders.

How to do a Kettlebell Squat

1. Stand tall with your feet shoulder-width apart and toes pointed outwards and hold the base of the kettlebell in both hands with palms facing each other.

2. Bend elbows and bring kettlebell up to the chest level with its handle facing you.

3. Squat downwards by bending both knees 90 degrees until your thighs are parallel with the floor and your hips drop below knees.

4. Stand back up and push hips forward as you stand up.

5. Squat downwards immediately.

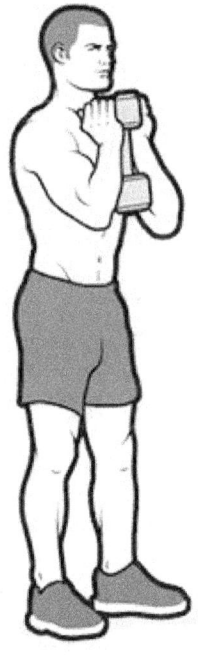
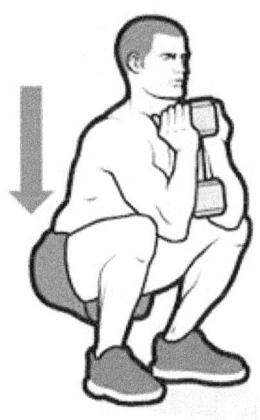

Tips to Perform Kettlebell Squat Correctly

Keep the kettlebell stable through the movement in front of your chest. Avoid bending the back and shoulders. Stand tall and do not let the knees bend inward.

Video: https://youtu.be/LNsI2Ugcu9s

Kettlebell Deadlift

Kettlebell Deadlift is a frightening name of an extremely functional kettlebell exercise that utilizes every muscle in your body, burns more calories, builds strength, increases flexibility and turn on your nervous system all at once. It strengthens the muscles of your back, hips, glutes, and hamstrings.

Like kettlebell squats, the kettlebell deadlift is one of the fundamental daily human movements. It is basically the action of lifting a weight off the ground. So, whenever you scoop up your kid in your arms or lift a box off the floor, you are basically performing a deadlift.

How to do a Kettlebell Deadlift

1. Stand with your feet shoulder-width apart and a kettlebell placed in-between your legs.

2. Bend knees, tighten your lower back, and lower down to pick up the kettlebell.

3. Keep your hips back and your knees behind the toes.

4. Pick up the kettlebell and stand up using the power of your legs.

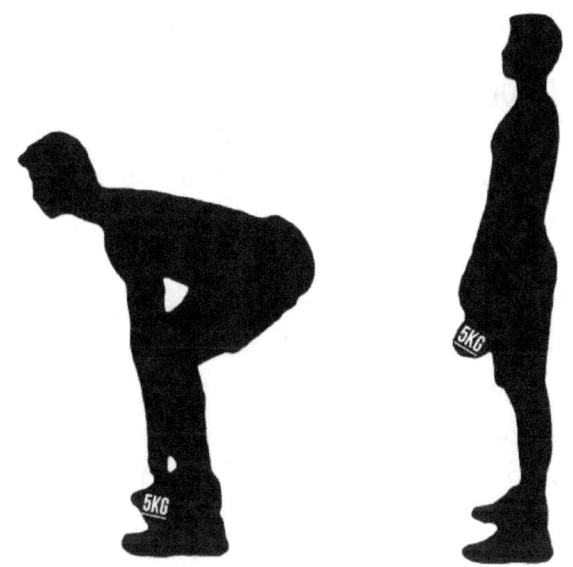

Tips to Perform Kettlebell Deadlift

In order to perform a kettlebell deadlift correctly you should keep your back flat, your hips above your knees, and your shins vertical.

Video: https://youtu.be/zF5CGQmNxyI

Variations of Kettlebell Deadlift

There are three variations of kettlebell deadlifts: single leg deadlift using single weight, single leg deadlift using two weights, and deadlift to squat thrust.

Single Leg Deadlift Using Single Weight

This variation of kettlebell deadlift is recommended for beginners. It is done using one kettlebell only. Using two kettlebells in the beginning of kettlebell training can lead to injury due to overextension. It is important to select an appropriate size of kettlebell to properly impact on your muscles.

Single Leg Deadlift Using Two Weights

Kettlebell deadlift with two weights is recommended for advanced lifters who have build enough strength after practicing kettlebell deadlifts with single weight.

Deadlift to Squat Thrust

This is one of the most intensive kettlebell exercises. It is a combination of kettlebell deadlift and squat thrust. It is done by bending downwards to the floor with a kettlebell in each hand. The legs are then moved forward in a single motion and the movement is finished off with a normal kettlebell deadlift.

Kettlebell Swing

Kettlebell swings are great full-body exercises for beginners that are designed to build strength and improve posture. The kettlebell swing is the basic of all ballistic kettlebell exercises. It is one of the most metabolic exercises that results in rapid calories burn and weight loss. It also increases strength of the shoulders and lower back.

Kettlebell swings are best for individuals who have back pain or other problems because of sedentary lifestyle. They are also very helpful in maintaining cardiovascular fitness. A study conducted by the U.S. Truman State University showed that traditional kettlebell swing is a more effective cardio workout than other traditional weight training circuits.

The kettlebell swing is one of the basic kettlebell exercises, which trains a beginner to perform hip hinges that are essential to perform advanced kettlebell exercises such as kettlebell deadlifts and all bent over rows.

How to do a Kettlebell Swing

1. Stand with your feet shoulder-length apart and hold a kettlebell with both hands.

2. Slightly bend your knees while keeping your chest lifted.

3. Push your hips backward and hinge your torso until it is parallel with the floor.

4. Extend your arms and allow the kettlebell to drop between your legs.

5. Squeeze your glutes and push hips forward

6. Propel the kettlebell to shoulder-height and allow it to swing back down.

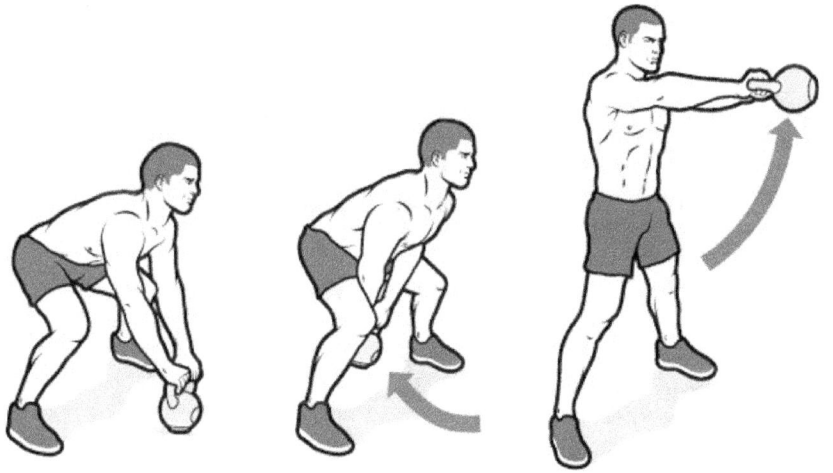

Tips to Perform a Kettlebell Swing Correctly

Make sure that your feet are planted firmly on the floor and shoulders are connected to the body. There should be no forward knee movement on the upswing and spine should be neutral. The back should be flat to avoid any injury.

Video: https://youtu.be/q0jalJ-3e7U

Kettlebell One-Handed Swing

Single-arm or one-handed kettlebell swing is a more intensive variation of the traditional kettlebell swing. It works the same way as the two-handed swing but is much more demanding on your whole body. It helps in developing a stronger midline and a stronger lower back through stabilization and activation of the core muscles. It strengthens the hamstrings and glutes. Kettlebell one-handed swing also improves cardiovascular endurance.

Kettlebell one-handed swing is performed the same way as the traditional kettlebell swing. The obvious difference is that it is performed with one hand instead of two.

How to do a Kettlebell One-Handed Swing

1. Place the kettlebell in front of you on the ground, settled in between your legs.

2. Stand straight with your head up, hips back, chest open, and weight on your heels.

3. Grasp the kettlebell with one hand and simultaneously extend your legs and pull the kettlebell up.

4. Your goal is to project the kettlebell to your chest level. It is normal to take few repetitions to get it to your chest or eye level.

5. Perform five to ten repetitions and then place the kettlebell back on the ground. Switch hands and perform kettlebell swings for five to ten times again.

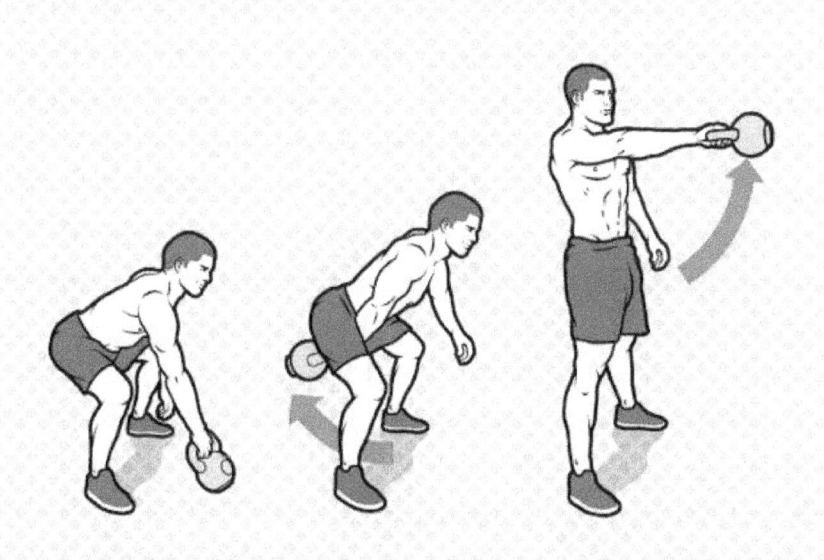

You can also attempt to do single-handed kettlebell swing with hand switch. The key in this movement is timing. Switch the kettlebell from one hand to another when it is at the top end of the swing.

Tips for Performing One-Handed Kettlebell Swings Correctly

The most important consideration in a kettlebell swing is your spine position. Any sort of flexion can be dangerous and cause injuries. Apply force only when extending your hips and legs.

Too much tension throughout the whole movement can reduce the efficiency and power of the exercise.

Video: https://youtu.be/9W7ZiimlfaE

Safety Tips for Kettlebell Training

Consistency with kettlebell training is the key to losing weight and getting fit quickly. Time spent away from kettlebell training due to wounds, or icing knees, shoulders, and wrists is a waste of time. You can get in shape by spending this time in burning fat of your body and building lean muscles. Therefore, it is best to take some safety measures and not get hurt in order to perform consistently and get quicker results.

Warm Up

Even if you are an advanced lifter and have been training with heavier kettlebells for months and years, it is always a good idea to do some push-ups, light stretching, and a few minutes of cardio before doing ballistic exercises with a heavy kettlebell. It is important to warm up in order to prevent any muscle pull or muscle spasm.

Quick 2 minute kettlebell warm up: https://youtu.be/QSYU-6EwPqI

Don't Push Yourself

It is good to set higher targets but do not push yourself to start kettlebell training with a 24kg kettlebell if you are a novice. Proceed step by step, practice with lighter kettlebells first, and master a technique before moving on to heavier kettlebells and intensive movements.

Breathe Properly

Proper breathing is essential for using a kettlebell safely. Concentrate on the technique rather than on the volume of repetitions. If you are doing an intensive movement such as a deadlift to squat thrust and you find yourself exhausted and breathless, take a moment and switch to lighter basic kettlebell movements to catch your breath.

Proper breathing is also important to minimize the pressure on your spine. Abdominal bracing is a technique, which utilizes breathing patterns to tighten the abdominal muscles that in turn protect your spine. Practice this technique to know how you can tighten your abdominal muscles as you exhale.

Eliminate Distractions

Kettlebell training requires focus and concentration. Distractions and interruptions not only decrease the effectiveness of kettlebell training, they increase the risk of injuries too. Focus on your technique and breathing instead of contemplating things that do not matter in that moment.

Choose the Right Size

Your wrong selection of kettlebell not only can hurt you but it can hurt others as well. Kettlebell training is very different from traditional weight lifting and cardio workout. It is wise to get help from an expert in selecting appropriate kettlebell for you. A kettlebell that is too heavy for your strength and ability can lead to an ineffective training session as well as injuries. It is better to start with a lighter kettlebell and master the basic techniques with it before moving up to a heavier kettlebell and intensive movements.

Beware of Your Surroundings

Always ensure that you have enough room around you to perform the movements without harming other people, objects, or yourself. Kettlebell training involves dynamic movements. Have a clear floor space with no object on the floor to trip over. Stay clear of wall and mirrors and anything else that can be harmed if you lose control of the kettlebell. Do not try to catch the kettlebell if you lose control or drop it during an exercise. Let it drop on the floor. The worst thing that can happen is that you damage the floor.

Learn the Technique

Learning proper kettlebell movements from an experienced instructor is essential. Improper positioning of the body can lead to injuries in the shoulders and back. Maintaining a firm grip on the kettlebell and wearing flat-soled shoes are two important considerations for all types of kettlebell exercises.

Do Not Stop Moving

Once you are done with your kettlebell training, do not stand still or sit down. Walk around the room until your heart rate and breathing normalize. Standing or sitting still immediately after kettlebell training can elevate blood pressure that can cause serious health complications.

Beginner Kettlebell Workouts.

Workout 1A - The Newbie

"In the beginner's mind there are many possibilities, but in the expert's there are few" - Shunryu Suzuki

If you have never used Kettlebells before I strongly suggest you do only this workout for the first couple of weeks while you get used to swinging the Kettlebell.

It's a nice easy workout that is designed to get you into Kettlebells slowly and help you get the functional movements down without

Time: 10 minutes (Split into 1 minute rounds)

Exercises: Two Handed Kettlebell Swing

Set a timer for 1 minute rounds and each minute you need to do 10 swings. If you feel any pain or discomfort end the workout immediately.

Minute 1: 10 two-handed swings

Minute 2: 10 two-handed swings

Minute 3: 10 two-handed swings

Minute 4: 10 two-handed swings

Minute 5: 10 swings

Minute 6: 10 swings

And so on until you have done 10 minutes (and 100 swings).

Workout 1B - The Bilbo Baggins

"It's a dangerous business, Frodo, going out of your door" - Bilbo Baggins

Yes stay in and do this Kettlebell workout instead. Much safer! This is where I begin to challenge you with the workouts and make you exhale a little (or a lot depending on your fitness level). But don't worry I haven't made it too difficult.

Time: 10 minutes (Split into 1 minute rounds)

Exercises: Two Handed Kettlebell Swing

Set a timer for 1 minute rounds and each minute you need to do the required number of swings. Once you have finished rest for the remainder of the round. If you feel any pain or discomfort end the workout immediately.

Minute 1: 20 two-handed swings

Minute 2: 20 two-handed swings

Minute 3: 20 two-handed swings

Minute 4: 20 two-handed swings

Minute 5: 20 two-handed swings

Minute 6: 20 two-handed swings

And so on until you have done the whole 10 minutes. You should have about 20-30 seconds rest between rounds after finishing your 20 swings. The quicker you get your 20 swings done the more rest you will get between rounds. Do not rush the exercises make sure to maintain proper form at all costs.

Workout 1C - The Jesse Pinkman

"This is my own private domicile and I will not be harassed...bitch" - Jesse Pinkman

Why go to a gym and be harassed by Personal Trainers? Stay home and get in shape instead. Gatorade me bitch!

Time: 10 minutes (Split into 1 minute rounds)

Exercises: Two Handed Kettlebell Swing

This is where the workouts start to get a little more challenging. By minute 5 you should be breathing heavy and by minute 9 you should be feeling tired.

Minute 1: 30 two-handed swings

Minute 2: 30 two-handed swings

Minute 3: 30 two-handed swings

Minute 4: 30 two-handed swings

Minute 5: 30 two-handed swings

Minute 6: 30 two-handed swings

And so on until you have done the whole 10 minutes. You should have about 20-30 seconds rest between rounds. As the workouts are picking up intensity it is really important to do 30 air squats to warm up and then some more to warm down at the end of the workout.

Intermediate Kettlebell Workouts.

Workout 2A - The Batman

"You either die a hero or live long enough to see yourself become the villain. " - Bruce Wayne

Stay in and do some kettlebells instead then you'll always be a hero.

Time: About 10 minutes

Exercises: Two Handed Kettlebell Swing, Kettlebell Squat

If you feel any pain or discomfort end the workout immediately.

20 Two Handed Kettlebell Swings

20 Kettlebell Squats

20 Two Handed Kettlebell Swings

20 Kettlebell Squats

20 Two Handed Kettlebell Swings

20 Kettlebell Squats

20 Two Handed Kettlebell Swings

20 Kettlebell Squats

20 Two Handed Kettlebell Swings

20 Kettlebell Squats

20 Two Handed Kettlebell Swings

20 Kettlebell Squats

Try to do the entire workout without resting. It will be hard if you need to have a rest take one, but try and get as far through the workout as you can before needing one. By the time you have finished you will have done 200 reps. Congratulate yourself. Make sure to always use proper form. Remember Batman always uses proper form!

Workout 2B - The Good, The Bad and The Ugly

"You see, in this world there's two kinds of people, my friend: Those with loaded guns and those who dig. You dig." - Blondie (1966)

Actually there's two kinds of people: those that swing and those who don't. You are a swinger. NO not that kind!!

Time: About 12 minutes

Exercises: Two Handed Kettlebell Swing, One Handed Kettlebell Swing

This is going to be the hardest workout so far

20 Two Handed Kettlebell Swings

10 Left-Hand Kettlebell Swings

10 Right-Hand Kettlebell Swings

20 Two Handed Kettlebell Swings

10 Left-Hand Kettlebell Swings

10 Right-Hand Kettlebell Swings

20 Two Handed Kettlebell Swings

10 Left-Hand Kettlebell Swings

10 Right-Hand Kettlebell Swings

20 Two Handed Kettlebell Swings

10 Left-Hand Kettlebell Swings

10 Right-Hand Kettlebell Swings

20 Two Handed Kettlebell Swings

10 Left-Hand Kettlebell Swings

10 Right-Hand Kettlebell Swings

So by the end you will have done 5 sets of 20 two-handed swings and 20 single handed swings (10 left and 10 right). 200 swings in total for the entire workout. Try and do as much of the workout as you can without resting. If you form starts to deteriorate make sure you rest for a minute or two.

Workout 2C - The Sterling Archer

"Call Kenny Loggins cause you're in the Danger Zone!" - Sterling Archer

All I've had today, is like six gummy bears and some scotch.

Time: About 10 minutes

Exercises: Two Handed Kettlebell Swing, Kettlebell Squat

If you feel any pain or discomfort end the workout immediately.

30 Two Handed Kettlebell Swings

20 Kettlebell Squats

30 Two Handed Kettlebell Swings

20 Kettlebell Squats

30 Two Handed Kettlebell Swings

20 Kettlebell Squats

30 Two Handed Kettlebell Swings

20 Kettlebell Squats

30 Two Handed Kettlebell Swings

20 Kettlebell Squats

30 Two Handed Kettlebell Swings

20 Kettlebell Squats

Try to do the entire workout without resting. It will be hard if you need to have a rest take one, but try and get as far through the workout as you can before needing one. By the time you have finished you will have done 200 reps. Congratulate yourself. Make sure to always use proper form. Batman always uses proper form!

Advanced Kettlebell Workouts.

Workout 3A - Darth Vader

"Impressive. Most impressive. Obi-Wan has taught you well. You have controlled your fear. Now, release your anger. Only your hatred can destroy me" - Darth Vader

Can't destroy you today, I'm too busy being awesome.

Time: About 10 minutes

Exercises: Two Handed Kettlebell Swing

If you feel any pain or discomfort end the workout immediately.

15 Seconds - 2 Handed Kettlebell Swings

15 Seconds - Rest

15 Seconds - 2 Handed Kettlebell Swings

15 Seconds - Rest

15 Seconds - 2 Handed Kettlebell Swings

15 Seconds - Rest

15 Seconds - 2 Handed Kettlebell Swings

15 Seconds - Rest

15 Seconds - 2 Handed Kettlebell Swings

15 Seconds - Rest

And so on until you have done 5 minutes of kettlebell swings. That will be 20 rounds of 15 seconds of swings and a 15 second rest. This is what is known as a HIIT workout (High Intensity Interval Training). This will undoubtedly get you breathing heavily and sweating. Due to the fat burning power of kettlebells paired with the fat burning power of HIIT workouts you will see a massive difference if you do this workout one or two times a week.

Workout 3B - The Superman

"You will give the people of Earth an ideal to strive towards. They will race behind you, they will stumble, they will fall. But in time, they will join you in the sun, Kal. In time, you will help them accomplish wonders. " - Jor-El

No need to go outside in your underwear do it from the comfort of your own home.

Time: About 10 minutes

Exercises: Two Handed Kettlebell Swing

If you feel any pain or discomfort end the workout immediately.

30 Seconds - 2 Handed Kettlebell Swings

30 Seconds - Rest

30 Seconds - 2 Handed Kettlebell Swings

30 Seconds - Rest

30 Seconds - 2 Handed Kettlebell Swings

30 Seconds - Rest

30 Seconds - 2 Handed Kettlebell Swings

30 Seconds - Rest

30 Seconds - 2 Handed Kettlebell Swings

30 Seconds - Rest

And so on until you have done 5 minutes of kettlebell swings. That will be 10 rounds of 30 seconds of swings and a 30 second rest. This workout will be significantly harder than the last one after about 6 rounds. You will feel like quitting but stay the course and keep going.

Workout 3C - Jon Snow

"You know nothing, Jon Snow." - Ygritte

He might not know nothing about most things but he knows that this workout is hard work.

Time: About 10 minutes

Exercises: Two Handed Kettlebell Swing

If you feel any pain or discomfort end the workout immediately.

60 Seconds - 2 Handed Kettlebell Swings

60 Seconds - Rest

60 Seconds - 2 Handed Kettlebell Swings

60 Seconds - Rest

60 Seconds - 2 Handed Kettlebell Swings

60 Seconds - Rest

60 Seconds - 2 Handed Kettlebell Swings

60 Seconds - Rest

60 Seconds - 2 Handed Kettlebell Swings

60 Seconds - Rest

And so on until you have done 5 minutes of kettlebell swings. That will be 5 rounds of 1 minute of swings and a 1 minute rest. This workout will be significantly harder than the last one after about 6 rounds. You arms will feel like lead weights by the halfway point of this workout.

The Iron Throne

"There is a savage beast in every man, and when you hand that man a sword or spear and send him forth to war, the beast stirs."

This is the brutal Kettlebell workout I have ever done. The Red Wedding has nothing on this!

Time: About 10 minutes

Exercises: Two Handed Kettlebell Swing, Two handed Kettlebell Squat

If you feel any pain or discomfort end the workout immediately.

60 Seconds - 2 Handed Kettlebell Swings

60 Seconds - Kettlebell Squat

60 Seconds - 2 Handed Kettlebell Swings

60 Seconds - Kettlebell Squat

60 Seconds - 2 Handed Kettlebell Swings

60 Seconds - Kettlebell Squat

60 Seconds - 2 Handed Kettlebell Swings

60 Seconds - Kettlebell Squat

60 Seconds - 2 Handed Kettlebell Swings

60 Seconds - Kettlebell Squat

And so on until you have done 5 minutes of kettlebell swings and kettlebell squats. That will be 5 rounds of 1 minute of swings and 1 minute of squats immediately after. This workout will mentally and physically break you. If you need a rest take one but try and go for as long as you can without needing it. You will need a long lie down after finishing. Congratulations you have made it to the hardest workout in the book.

Conclusion

Now you know how to Supercharge your workout to lose fat and get into great shape fast in as little time possible. Give the workout in this book a try for a month or so and I guarantee you'll see better results than if you were to do the traditional long, slow cardio workouts using fitness equipment at your gym. You'll lose belly fat, build a bit of lean muscle, look better, and have more fun too.

Remember that diet is important too. By cutting back on carbohydrates or following a high protein diet (such as the Paleo Diet) you'll see results even faster.

www.ingramcontent.com/pod-product-compliance
Lightning Source LLC
Chambersburg PA
CBHW070230290526
45789CB00004B/1565